DIABETES DIET

A Total Diet Guide For People With Diabetes.

KELVIN BRYAN

Table of Contents

CHAPTER ONE

INTRODUCTION

A diabetes food regimen virtually means eating the healthiest foods in moderate quantities and sticking to ordinary mealtimes.

A diabetes food regimen is a wholesome-eating plan that's clearly rich in nutrients and coffee in fat and energy. Key factors are fruits, greens and whole grains. In truth, a diabetes weight-reduction plan is the best ingesting plan for maximum all of us.

When you have diabetes or prediabetes, your doctor will in all likelihood advice that you see a dietitian to help you expand a healthy-consuming plan. The plan facilitates you manipulate your blood sugar (glucose), control your weight and control heart sickness hazard elements, including excessive blood pressure and high blood fats.

Whilst you consume greater energy and fat, your frame creates an undesirable rise in blood glucose. If blood glucose is not saved in check, it can result in severe problems, which include a excessive blood glucose level (hyperglycemia) that, if continual, may additionally cause lengthy-term complications, along with nerve, kidney and heart harm.

You can help keep your blood glucose degree in a safe variety via making healthy food alternatives and tracking your consuming behavior.

For the majority with type 2 diabetes, weight loss can also make it easier to manipulate blood glucose and offers a host of different fitness benefits. In case you need to lose weight, a diabetes food plan offers a properly-prepared, nutritious manner to attain your goal correctly.

CHAPTER TWO

OVERVIEW OF DIABETES DIET

A diabetes eating regimen is primarily based on eating 3 meals an afternoon at ordinary times. This facilitates you better use the insulin that your frame produces or gets thru a medicine.

A registered dietitian allows you to put together a diet primarily based in your health desires, tastes and way of life. She or he can also talk with you approximately the way to improve your ingesting habits, such as deciding on portion sizes that fit the needs in your length and interest stage.

Recommended Ingredients

Make your energy depend with these nutritious meals. Choose healthful carbohydrates, fiber-rich meals, fish and "appropriate" fat.

Healthy carbohydrates

All through digestion, sugars (simple carbohydrates) and starches (complex carbohydrates) destroy down into blood glucose.

Recognition on wholesome carbohydrates, together with:

•   Culmination

•   Greens

•   Whole grains

•   Legumes, inclusive of beans and peas

•   Low-fats dairy products, which include milk and cheese. Avoid less healthy carbohydrates, inclusive of foods or beverages with brought fat, sugars and sodium.

Fiber-rich ingredients

Nutritional fiber includes all elements of plant foods that your frame cannot digest or soak up. Fiber moderates how your body digests and allows manipulate blood sugar levels. Foods high in fiber encompass:

- Veggies

- End result

- Nuts

- Legumes, which includes beans and peas

- Entire grains

Coronary heart-wholesome fish

Eat heart-healthful fish at the least twice a week. Fish which includes salmon, mackerel, tuna and sardines are wealthy in omega-3 fatty acids, which can also save you heart disorder.

Keep away from fried fish and fish with excessive stages of mercury, such as king mackerel.

Appropriate fat

Foods containing monounsaturated and polyunsaturated fat can help decrease your cholesterol levels. These include:

- Avocados

- Nuts

- Canola, olive and peanut oils

However do not overdo it, as all fats are excessive in energy.

CHAPTER THREE

FOODS TO AVOID

Diabetes will increase your risk of heart sickness and stroke through accelerating the development of clogged and hardened arteries. Foods containing the following can work in opposition to your intention of a heart-healthful weight loss plan.

• Saturated fats. Avoid high-fats dairy merchandise and animal proteins consisting of butter, red meat, hot puppies, sausage and also limit coconut and palm kernel oils.

•   Trans fat. Avoid trans fats located in processed snacks, baked goods, shortening and stick margarines.

•   LDL cholesterol. LDL cholesterol assets encompass excessive-fat dairy merchandise and excessive-fats animal proteins, egg yolks, liver and other organ meats. Aim for no greater than two hundred milligrams (mg) of LDL cholesterol an afternoon.

•   Sodium. Aim for less than 2,300 mg of sodium a day. Your physician can also advise you intention for even less when you have excessive blood stress.

You may use a few unique procedures to create a diabetes weight-reduction plan that will help you maintain your blood glucose stage inside a normal variety. With a dietitian's assist, you may find that one or an aggregate of the subsequent methods works for you:

The plate approach

The yank Diabetes association gives an easy method of meal planning. In essence, it makes a specialty of consuming extra greens. Comply with these steps whilst preparing your plate:

• Fill 1/2 of your plate with nonstarchy vegetables, together with spinach, carrots and tomatoes.

• Fill 1 / 4 of your plate with a protein, consisting of tuna, lean beef or bird.

• Fill the remaining area with a whole-grain object, consisting of brown rice, or a starchy vegetable, such as inexperienced peas.

• encompass "excellent" fat including nuts or avocados in small amounts.

- upload a serving of fruit or dairy and a drink of water or unsweetened tea or coffee.

Counting carbohydrates

Because carbohydrates break down into glucose, they have the best effect in your blood glucose stage. To assist manipulate your blood sugar, you could need to learn how to calculate the quantity of carbohydrates you are eating so that you can modify the dose of insulin for this reason. It's important to hold music of the quantity of carbohydrates in every meal or snack.

A dietitian can educate you the way to measure food quantities and end up an educated reader of food labels. She or he also can train you the way to pay special interest to serving size and carbohydrate content material.

In case you're taking insulin, a dietitian can train you how to count number the amount of carbohydrates in each meal or snack and alter your insulin dose therefore.

CHAPTER FOUR

HOW TO PICK YOUR MEALS

A dietitian may additionally recommend you pick out particular meals that will help you plan food and snacks. You can choose a number of foods from lists together with classes inclusive of carbohydrates, proteins and fats.

One serving in a class is known as a "desire." A meals desire has approximately the same quantity of carbohydrates, protein, fat and calories — and the same effect to your blood glucose — as a serving of every other food in that same class. As an example, the starch, fruits and milk listing consists of selections that are 12 to 15 grams of carbohydrates.

A few humans who have diabetes use the glycemic index to select foods, in particular carbohydrates. This method ranks carbohydrate-containing ingredients primarily based on their effect on blood glucose stages. Talk with your dietitian about whether this technique would possibly give you the results you want.

A pattern menu

Whilst planning meals, recall your length and hobby stage.

• Breakfast. Whole-wheat bread (1 medium slice) with 2 teaspoons jelly, 1/2 cup shredded wheat cereal with a cup of one percent low-fat milk, a bit of fruit, coffee

• Lunch. Roast red meat sandwich on wheat bread with lettuce, low-fat American cheese, tomato and mayonnaise, medium apple, water

• Dinner. Salmon, 1 1/2 of teaspoons vegetable oil, small

baked potato, half cup carrots, 1/2 cup inexperienced beans, medium white dinner roll, unsweetened iced tea, milk

- Snack. 2 1/2 cups popcorn with 1 1/2 teaspoons margarine

What are the results of a diabetes food regimen?

Embracing your healthful-eating plan is the first-rate way to maintain your blood glucose stage below manages and save you diabetes headaches. And if you need to lose weight, you could tailor it on your unique desires.

Aside from handling your diabetes, a diabetes food regimen offers different blessings, too. Because a diabetes eating regimen recommends beneficent amounts of end result, veggies and fiber, following it's far in all likelihood to reduce your hazard of cardiovascular diseases and positive varieties of most cancers. And eating low-fats dairy merchandise can lessen your danger of low bone mass within the destiny.

CHAPTER FIVE

FATTY FISH AS DIABETES DIET

Fatty fish is one of the healthiest ingredients in the world.

Salmon, sardines, herring, anchovies and mackerel are exceptional sources of the omega-3 fatty acids DHA and EPA, which have important advantages for heart fitness.

Getting enough of these fats on a normal foundation is specially critical for diabetics, who've a multiplied hazard of heart ailment and stroke.

DHA and EPA defend the cells that line your blood vessels, lessen markers of inflammation and enhance the manner your arteries function after eating.

A number of observational studies advocate that individuals who eat fatty fish regularly have a decrease hazard of heart failure and are much less possibly to die from heart disease.

In studies, older males and females who fed on fatty fish five–7 days per week for eight weeks had large reductions in triglycerides and inflammatory markers.

Fatty fish comprise omega-three fats that reduce irritation and different risk elements for heart sickness and stroke.

CHAPTER SIX

LEAFY VEGGIES AND CHIA SEEDS

Leafy veggies

Leafy inexperienced greens are extraordinarily nutritious and coffee in energy.

They're additionally very low in digestible carbs, which raise your blood sugar levels.

Spinach, kale and different leafy greens are proper assets of several nutrients and minerals, consisting of nutrition C.

In a single observe, growing diet C intake decreased inflammatory markers and fasting blood sugar ranges for humans with type 2 diabetes or high blood pressure. Similarly, leafy greens are right assets of the antioxidants lutein and zeaxanthin.

These antioxidants protect your eyes from macular degeneration and cataracts that are common diabetes headaches.

Leafy green greens are rich in vitamins and antioxidants that guard your coronary heart and eye health.

Eggs

Eggs offer notable fitness blessings.

In reality, they're one of the high-quality foods for maintaining you complete for hours.

Ordinary egg consumption might also lessen your coronary heart disease danger in numerous approaches.

Eggs lower irritation, improve insulin sensitivity, increase your "exact" HDL cholesterol levels and alter the scale and form of your "terrible" LDL cholesterol.

In a single examine, human beings with type 2 diabetes who fed on 2 eggs day by day as part of a high-protein diet had upgrades in LDL cholesterol and blood sugar stages.

Similarly, eggs are one of the first-rate sources of lutein and zeaxanthin, antioxidants that protect the eyes from sickness.

Simply make sure to devour entire eggs. The benefits of eggs are typically because of nutrients discovered in the yolk as opposed to the white.

Eggs enhance risk elements for heart sickness, sell excellent blood sugar control, guard eye fitness and maintain you feeling complete.

Chia seeds

Chia seeds are a top notch food for humans with diabetes.

They're extremely excessive in fiber, yet low in digestible carbs.

In reality, 11 of the 12 grams of carbs in a 28-gram (1-ounces) serving of chia seeds are fiber, which doesn't enhance blood sugar.

The viscous fiber in chia seeds can virtually decrease your blood sugar tiers by using slowing down the rate at which meals movements via your gut and is absorbed.

Chia seeds may also assist you gain a healthful weight because fiber reduces starvation and makes you experience complete. In addition, fiber can decrease the quantity of energy you soak up from other meals eaten on the same meal.

Moreover, chia seeds have been proven to lessen blood strain and inflammatory markers.

Chia seeds contain high quantities of fiber, are low in digestible carbs and can lower blood pressure and irritation.

Turmeric

Turmeric is a spice with powerful fitness advantages.

Its active aspect, curcumin, can lower inflammation and blood sugar levels, at the same time as decreasing coronary heart disease risk.

What's extra, curcumin appears to advantage kidney fitness in diabetics. That is critical, as diabetes is one of the main causes of kidney disorder.

Lamentably, curcumin isn't absorbed that properly on its own. Make certain to devour turmeric with piperine (discovered in black pepper) that allows you to improve absorption with the aid of as a good deal as 2,000%.

Turmeric incorporates curcumin, which can also reduce blood sugar stages and inflammation, even as protecting against heart and kidney disease.

Greek Yogurt

Greek yogurt is a super dairy desire for diabetics.

It's been proven to enhance blood sugar control and decrease coronary heart disease hazard, possibly in part because of the probiotics it include.

Studies have determined that yogurt and other dairy ingredients may also result in weight loss and advanced frame composition in people with type 2 diabetes.

It's believed that dairy's high calcium and conjugated linolic acid (CLA) content may additionally play a role.

What's greater, Greek yogurt includes most effective 6–8 grams of carbs according to serving, which is decrease than traditional yogurt. It's additionally better in protein, which promotes weight loss with the aid of lowering appetite and reducing calorie consumption.

Greek yogurt promotes healthy blood sugar stages, reduces danger elements for coronary heart disorder and might help with weight management. Nuts

Nuts are scrumptious and nutritious.

All sorts of nuts comprise fiber and are low in digestible carbs, although some have greater than others.

Here are the amounts of digestible carbs in step with 1-oz. (28-gram) serving of nuts:

- Almonds: 2.6 grams

- Brazil nuts: 1.4 grams

- Cashews: 7.7 grams

- Hazelnuts: 2 grams

- Macadamia: 1.5 grams

- Pecans: 1.2 grams

- Pistachios: 5 grams

- Walnuts: 2 grams

Research on a ramification of various nuts has proven that ordinary intake may additionally reduce inflammation and lower blood sugar, HbA1c and LDL tiers.

In a single look at, human beings with diabetes who protected 30 grams of walnuts in their day by day food regimen for 365 days misplaced weight, had improvements in frame composition and experienced a big discount in insulin ranges.

This finding is important due to the fact human beings with kind 2 diabetes often have accelerated degrees of insulin, which are related to weight problems.

further, a few researchers accept as true with chronically excessive insulin ranges boom the chance of other extreme illnesses, together with cancer and Alzheimer's ailment.

THANK YOU

www.ingramcontent.com/pod-product-compliance
Lightning Source LLC
Chambersburg PA
CBHW051405150726
48000CB00003B/1345